The Art of Healing

~Physical/Nutrition ~
Mental/Mind ~

Copyright © 2023
ISBN: **ISBN:** 9798862496208

Whole Foods 4 Healthy Living

The Art of Healing

This book is intended to provide information and motivation to our readers. The content is the sole expression and opinion of its author, and not necessarily that of the publisher. No warranties or guarantees are expressed or implied by the publisher's choice to include any of the content in this volume. Neither the publisher nor the individual author(s) shall be liable for any physical, psychological, emotional, financial, or commercial damages, including, but not limited to, special, incidental, consequential or other damages. Our views and rights are the same: You are responsible for your own choices, actions, and results.

The Art of Healing

Author: Skip Stein

Table of Contents

The Art of Healing

The Art of Healing

The Art of Healing

The Art of Healing has been known for Centuries to be a complex process that often involves simple approaches that have been proven to be highly effective. The process begins with a diagnostic approach that is often begun with the patient's observable symptoms. But these symptoms often reveal a deeper causality in their expression besides the physical manifestation.

Today's medical approach is usually focused on the observable symptoms; the doctor treats the symptoms without ever exploring the foundation/basis of the expression of those symptoms. The goal is to treat the symptom, but not cure the patient of the ailment that is expressing the symptoms. So called 'modern medicine' is a one-legged stool that is bound to eventually collapse because it only treats symptoms and not the foundation or source of expression of the symptoms.

The Art of Healing

Healing is a much more complex process and must address more than just a symptomatic reduction. There is always a foundational cause of the symptom being expressed and this can often be a complex mixture of the physical, psychological and metaphysical expression of the human being treated.

Expression of Symptoms

The physical manifestation of a symptom is usually complex and involves many potential aspects of the human physical body. This manifestation of a symptom can itself be caused by physical injury, disease or mental malfunction that itself can be caused by various trauma. In many cases these symptoms are brought out by an imbalance in the human body; either psychological or biological or a combination of both. Discounting obvious trauma from accidental injury this malfunction, as expressed by the symptom(s), are expressed in, what is termed, a disease. This can be anything from simple acne in teenagers or a common cold to more serious diabetes 2, cancer and heart/arterial disease and more. It is a complex dictionary of a multitude of ailments in this disease category and ALL are an unnatural condition of the human body.

If we first assume that the human body is a complex mechanism of interacting systems designed to be in perfect balance, then we can search for an imbalance in one or more of these systems that has been expressed by the symptom(s).

Beyond this interaction of systems of the human body, we must recognize that this human body is also a storage locker for trillions of microbial cells/organisms called the Micro-Biome. These microbes cover your body, inhabit your intestines and thrive in your lower gut! These little buggers work to make up more than 70% of

The Art of Healing

your Natural Immune System and mostly thrive in your gut on the fiber you consume.

All these microbes consist of more than two and a half (2.5) million microbial genes. These inhabit your brain, your intestines and organs and surface of your skin. In your nose, lungs and blood; literally everywhere. Science is still trying to figure it out, but in the meantime refer to this conglomeration of organisms to as the Micro-Biome.

This micro-biome is in constant interaction with the systems of the human body; communicating in a complex electro-chemical system that supports what we refer to as a Human Being. When one or more of these symptoms or symbiotic relationships are out of balance, the human body will express this imbalance by one or more symptoms and that is what we most often to refer to as disease or illness.

The Art of Healing

The Systems of the Human Body

The complex systems of the human body and each of their interaction with the micro-biome is little understood. In fact, this interaction is barely understood and only has begun being studied beginning around 2006 by teams in the USA, Canada, India, China, Russia and more.

The major system of the human body include:

Circulatory System/Cardiovascular System

Circulates blood around the body via the heart, arteries and veins,
delivering oxygen and nutrients to organs and cells and carrying their waste products away, as well as keeping the body's temperature in a safe range.

Digestive System/Excretory System

System to absorb nutrients and remove waste via the gastrointestinal tract, including
the mouth, esophagus, stomach and intestines.

Endocrine System

Influences the function of the body using hormones,

Integumentary System/Exocrine System

System that comprises skin, hair, nails, and sweat and other exocrine glands.

Immune System/Lymphatic System

Defends the body against pathogens that may harm the body. The system contains a network of lymphatic vessels that carry a clear fluid called lymph.

Muscular System

The Art of Healing

Enables the body to move using muscles.

Nervous System

Collects and processes information from the senses via nerves and the brain and tells the muscles to contract to cause physical actions.

Urinary System/Renal System

The Urinary system (also known as Renal System) filter blood with the help of kidneys to produce urine, and get rid of waste.

Reproductive System

The reproductive organs required for the production of offspring.

Respiratory System

Brings air into and out of the lungs to absorb oxygen and remove carbon dioxide.

The Art of Healing

Skeletal System

Bones maintain the structure of the body and its organs.

Each and every one of these systems represent a set of highly complex functions that interact with each and every other system of the human body. Now add in the complex interaction of the body's micro-biome that also communicates and interacts with each of these systems and you only begin to comprehend what it means to be a Human Being.

Now this is how a typical doctor views the human patient and the domain of the symptomology they try to return to a synergistic balance. But you may have noticed that, while the nervous system is mentioned, the brain and its complex interaction with all of the previously mentioned systems and micro-biome is missing. That is where we must go next!

The Art of Healing

The Art of Healing

The Human Mind

The human brain is often simply viewed as what is located inside the human head. This impossibly complex instrument is not only a physical component of the human body but exhibits electro-chemical interactions with every other human body system as well as the micro-biome. While many of these interactions are termed autonomic, the human brain is the ultimate control over each and every control component and interaction of these systems and yes, even with the micro-biome.

While many consider the brain the seat or core of the Human Mind, it goes much further and represents a significantly much more complex interaction with both the internal systems, micro-biome and the brain than anyone has yet to fully comprehend.

The mind is that which thinks, imagines, remembers, wills, and senses, and is the set

The Art of Healing

of faculties responsible for such phenomena. The mind is also associated with experiencing perception, pleasure and pain, belief, desire, intention, and emotion. The mind can include conscious and non-conscious states as well as sensory and non-sensory experiences.

In addition, the human mind can exercise control over each and every physical system in the human body via the mind-brain interface and may indeed interact with the micro-biome in as yet undiscovered ways.

The disciplines of psychology, philosophy and neuroscience all have attempted to understand, map and control the complexities of the human mind and its interactions for centuries. Yet still struggle to even begin to understand or comprehend what the human mind truly is.

The Art of Healing

The Gestalt of Being a Human Being

The gestalt of being a human being is not yet complete. This gestalt is a collection of physical, biological, psychological and symbiotic entities that creates a unified concept, configuration or pattern which is greater than the sum of its parts personality, or being. We really cannot call it a complete summation! We have yet to delve into the metaphysical aspects of the human mind-body systems interactions.

Many like to think of metaphysics as dealing with the basic questions of life, such as the relationship of man, mind, and the universe, which leads to answers to the age-old questions of anyone who has truly paused to reflect on life by asking the most fundamental questions of all – "who am I; what am I; where have I been, and where am I going?"

The Art of Healing

While I cannot answer these questions, they often have a direct impact of the symptomology of the human subject seeking treatment.

The expression of system imbalance can be caused by the mind or mental perception of a problem as experienced or being experienced by the patient. The initiation of these expressions of this system imbalance is commonly referred to as a symptom. So, we have come full circle: Physical, Mental & Metaphysical.

The Art of Healing

Restoration of Balance

Now that we have defined what symptomology is, and the multitude of complex interactions that manifest a system or set of systems of imbalances, we can begin to delve into the methods and ways to restore the systems balance of the human body and the restoration of the gestalt that the Human Being truly is.

In order to do so, this restoration must trace back from the expressed symptom(s) to the system or component expressing the symptom. This is the search for causality or trigger that unbalanced the perfect balance that is called Health. In so doing we will look into the Physical, Nutritional, Mental and Cognitive functions that impacts the physical and metaphysical aspect of how the human body exists in the day-to-day world.

While this writing is in no way intended to be a complete resolution to the ultimate problems of health, it is intended to point out the linkages and interactions that the human body's systems represent that is necessary to truly restore the human body to the perfect balance we refer to as Health.

Mental Health

This subject has been at issue for centuries and cannot be fully covered here. But we will point out the mental health or balanced mental processes can only be achieved in a human body that is well balance, physically, nutritionally and where each system is in synchronicity.

Mental issues may be initiated by a failure in any system process. Poor nutrition may cause an imbalance in the hormones that interact and are interacted upon by other bodily processes or functions. Often at the core is poor nutrition is what causes an imbalance of hormones and nutrition that feeds the human brain. This electro-chemical malfunction can be represented in a multitude of mental health issues and more are being discovered.

Physical and/or emotional stress, over exertion, and again poor nutrition that fails to nurture the body/brain system.

Power of Belief

The human mind is so powerful that it can control many human physical systems, often complicating the diagnosis or root cause of a disease. Often overlooked is this power of the human mind when it comes to curative factors that have been shown to overcome physical imbalance of systems by simply believing that a cure is possible.

Psychosomatic disorders refer to physical symptoms that may be manifested by mental factors. In a psychosomatic illness, emotional stress or other psychological problems play key roles in the course of the physical signs and symptoms. Poor nutrition/diet can cause stress that may be manifested in psychological or psychosomatic symptomology.

At the same time, the placebo effect can demonstrate the impact of symptom relief by the patient believing that a treatment, or sugar pill has curative properties; thus, bringing about the reversal of negative systems that were previously unbalanced.

Interestingly enough, there is little difference in the end result of restoration of patient health. The results are the same! Which is the better approach? Or is a combination better added to the portfolio of possibilities?

The patient who believes the 'doctor' and his prognosis can be their worst enemy when it comes to healing. Too many 'doctors' or therapists tell a patient that they are deadly ill and if the patient believes them, it may become a self-fulfilling prophecy.

The Art of Healing

The medical establishment has profited for decades from the process of telling the patient that they are deadly ill and that only a certain treatment or drug/chemical can help relieve the symptoms but never totally remove the ailment/disease. This perpetuates the care and guarantees the revenue stream for the doctor or medical institution.

The Art of Healing

Alternative Treatments

Usually actively ignored and disparaged by most of the traditional medical community are the vast range of alternative approaches to health and symptom reversal and the regaining of patient health offered by Nutrition and Alternative Treatment Therapists.

Just a few of these alternative therapies that may address the physical, metaphysical, mental and nutritional health of the patient include:

Acupuncture, Acupressure & Reflexology

Reflexology involves applying pressure to specific areas on the feet, hands, or ears. Much like acupuncture & acupressure these pressure points correspond to different body organs and systems. Pressing them is believed to positively affect these organs and a person's overall health.

The Art of Healing

Chinese medicine calls the energy that flows through your body qi. Chinese medicine practitioners believe qi disruptions create imbalances in your body's energy. Meridians are channels that carry life energy (qi or ch'i) throughout the body. The reasoning holds that illness can occur when one of these meridians is blocked or out of balance.

Some forms of acupuncture aim to rebalance qi with needles or pressure applied to points (acupoints) throughout your body. There are hundreds of these acupoints in your body along 14 major meridians. When needles are used, the patient is then left for some time to meditate or rest as the body realigns the body's energy flow.

Acupuncture treatments are often complimented by massage therapy that may combine acupressure therapy while offering therapeutic massage that can relieve stress, help relax muscles and offer general overall relaxation.

Chiropractic

Chiropractors use hands-on spinal manipulation and other realignment treatments. Proper alignment of the body's musculoskeletal structure, particularly the spine, will enable the body to heal itself without surgery or medication.

Manipulation is used to restore mobility to joints restricted by tissue injury caused by a traumatic event, such as falling, or repetitive stress.

The treatment plan may involve one or more manual adjustments in which the doctor manipulates the joints, using a controlled, sudden force to improve range and quality of motion. Many chiropractors also incorporate nutritional counseling and exercise/rehabilitation into the treatment plan. The goals of chiropractic care include the restoration of function and prevention of injury in addition to pain relief.

Tai Chi, Qigong & Yoga

Tai Chi, Qigong and Yoga share a long list of health and wellness benefits. Both can improve your balance, flexibility, strength, mobility, mood, quality of life, range of motion, reflexes, and thinking skills.

Tai Chi, Qigong and Yoga involve gentle, low-impact exercise to help improve your strength and balance, and both include an emphasis on meditation to promote spiritual wellness.

As with Yoga, Tai Chi and Qigong focuses on deep breathing and relaxation techniques, and it has been proven to reduce stress, enhancing your overall mental, physical, and spiritual wellbeing.

Unlike other alternative approaches both Tai Chi, Qigong and Yoga teach meditative and breathing disciplines that help relax, calm and provide a curative environment for the human body.

While very similar in practice the roots of each of these disciplines combine a slightly different metaphysical approach and belief system.

Electrotherapy

Electrotherapy is the use of electrical energy as a medical treatment. In medicine, the term electrotherapy can apply to a variety of treatments, including the use of electrical devices such as deep brain stimulators for neurological disease. The term has also been applied specifically to the use of electric current to speed wound healing. Additionally, the term "electrotherapy" or "electromagnetic therapy" has also been applied to a range of alternative medical devices and treatments.

The Art of Healing

Electrotherapy is typically used in conjunction with other treatments, rather than by itself. For people undergoing physical therapy, electrotherapy may alleviate pain sufficiently for an individual to participate more actively in targeted exercises. Electrotherapy is among pain relief options gaining attention as the potential risks and side effects of opioid (narcotic) medications have become more apparent.

Efforts to use electrical current to aid in healing go back to ancient times. The modern era of electrotherapy in the United States began with treatment for anxiety and depression, and the number of potential uses has grown since. Electrotherapy has been used to address chronic pain, chronic fatigue, fibromyalgia, migraine headaches and more.

The Art of Healing

Bioresonance

Bioresonance therapy is based on the concept that unhealthy cells or organs emit altered electromagnetic oscillations due to DNA damage, diseased organs and cancer cells. Theses electromagnetic oscillations vary from those emitted by healthy cells due to their differences in cell metabolism.

Proponents of bioresonance believe that detection of these waves can be used to diagnose disease, while changing these waves back to their normal frequency will treat disease.

To use bioresonance, electrodes are placed on the skin to detect and analyze the energy wavelengths coming from the body. The energy frequencies can be manipulated by the machine to allow the body's cells to vibrate at their "natural frequency," which may treat the condition.

Frequency Therapeutics

Albert Einstein once said, "Everything in life is vibration". Every atom has its own vibrational frequency, meaning they vibrate at varying rates. As humans, we also have a vibrational frequency.

Nikola Tesla said: "If you want to find the secrets of the universe, think in terms of energy, frequency and vibration."

Every human organism as well as every pathogen emits certain frequencies, frequency therapy is intended to vibrate the pathogens in such a way that they can be destroyed or weakened so the natural immune system can destroy them.

These frequencies can be measured in Hertz (Hz). For human beings, it is thought that a healthy frequency level falls in the range of 62-72 Hz. If a person's frequency level drops below 62 Hz, they are at a higher risk of disease and illness.

Frequency therapy is considered to be an alternative method of treatment, which brings amazing results not only in cancer, but also in a variety of other diseases.

In combination with the appropriate nutritional supplements, frequency therapy not only specifically kill pathogens, bacteria, fungi or viruses, but also support human organ functions, stimulate detoxification processes and strengthens the immune system.

Many musical compositions align well with Tesla's healing frequencies of 432 Hz you may well want to explore them as they are plentiful from many sources. We often play various ones for meditation and for sleep at night.

The Art of Healing

Homeopathy

Homeopathy is based on the principle of treating "like with like," meaning a substance that causes adverse reactions when taken in large doses can be used — in small amounts — to treat those same symptoms.

Homeopathy, also known as homeopathic medicine, is a medical system that was developed in Germany more than 200 years ago. It's based on two unconventional theories:

1. "Like cures like"—the notion that a disease can be cured by a substance that produces similar symptoms in healthy people.
2. "Law of minimum dose"—the concept that the lower the dose of the medication, the greater its effectiveness. Many homeopathic products are so

diluted that no molecules of the original substance remain.

Homeopathic products come from plants (such as red onion, arnica [mountain herb], poison ivy, belladonna [deadly nightshade], and stinging nettle), minerals (such as white arsenic), or animals (such as crushed whole bees). Homeopathic products are often made as sugar pellets to be placed under the tongue; they may also be in other forms, such as ointments, gels, drops, creams, and tablets.

Treatments are "individualized" or tailored to each person—it's common for different people with the same condition to receive different treatments. Homeopathy uses a different diagnostic system for assigning treatments to individuals and recognizes clinical patterns of signs and symptoms that are different from those of conventional medicine.

The Art of Healing

Power of Nutrition

Neglected and often actively rejected by most medical practitioners comes Nutrition and the foods we consume on a daily basis. These foodstuffs are what make up the human body, for good or for worse. In modern America, it is usually the latter.

Nutritional therapies cover a wide-ranging area of health approaches. While there are many theories and yes, quackeries, out there a few basic disciplines have proven effective and beneficial over the decades, and yes centuries.

Standard American Diet (SAD)

As long as America and much of the rest of the Planet continues to make poor food choices, we will ALWAYS be victims of the next 'pandemic'. The unfortunate World has followed the horrible dietary guides of a Standard American Diet for decades and this has resulted in a pandemic of chronic disease that would be both preventable and reversable IFF proper nutrition was considered. Few medical caregivers actually even mentioning nutrition and how it can maintain a healthy, strong, natural immune system that fights viruses and infectious crap all day, every day.

The Human Being has evolved (or been designed) with a miraculous natural immune system that combats the onslaught of germs, viruses and contagions that we come into contact with every hour of every day. No amount of cleaning, wearing masks or anything is as effective as your healthy natural immune system.

Unfortunately, too many follow a Standard American Deadly Diet of processed foods, fast food joints and eat no-fiber animal products instead of eating delicious natural whole foods; high in fiber and nutrition that feeds and maintains your natural immune system. But you will never hear this from

The Art of Healing

the talking heads controlled by big pharma and the medical industry who make billion$ from treating people to death. A medical industry, controlled by Major Corporations that manufacture patentable crap that, more often than not, have horrendous side effects, while claiming to treat the symptoms but never seem to actually cure anyone of the disease/ailment.

Chemical, genetic engineering and now bio-engineering of processed foods has been going on for many decades. They are nothing but drug pushers in lab coats who get kids addicted to this processed 'food' crap at an early age and this is part of the reason Americans and others are fat, sick and nearly dead.

This unnatural stuff destroys your Natural Immune System and makes you an easy prey for viruses, germs and other invaders. If we learn to focus on nutrition and not drugs, we will be healthier, happier and wiser. Living longer healthy, vibrant lives; not tied to a bedframe with tubes and wires; but out hiking/walking and enjoying our planetary wonders.

Now that we have presented the SAD way of eating that most Americans practice, lets also consider the lack of daily exercise that many/most Americans fail to achieve. This only compounds the exposure to illness that most Americans face and further makes them susceptible to illness.

Natural Whole Food Lifestylediet

Webster's Dictionary has 4 variations of meaning for the word 'diet'. One is food and drink regularly consumed. Two is habitual nourishment. Three is the kind and amount of food prescribed for a specific reason (goal). Fourth is a regimen of eating and drinking sparingly so as to reduce one's weight. All these refer to eating food but has no definition of what types of food are to be consumed. So, the word 'diet' is pretty much up for grabs by anyone who wants to use it to apply to a way of consuming food.

What you eat regularly in the first use is more relevant to how you live and consume nourishment to stay alive. Diet seems to define the necessary nourishment to provide nutrients required by our bodies to survive, do work and live/exist in a healthy active format. I prefer to call this *lifestyle*; but that too can be confusing.

Lifestyle is defined as a typical way of life or living for an individual, group or culture. Wow, culture, in the aspect of eating or food opens up a Pandora's Box of alternatives by itself. How does 'diet' pertain to a cultural way of eating; such diversity and variations in choices, selections and regional/climatological variations. What a cultural group eats to survive depends on

The Art of Healing

location, availability and climate; what is available as a food source.

We are really getting into the weeds, so to speak, here. I'm getting confused writing this! Defining what we eat on a regular/daily basis involves both diet and lifestyle. Lifestyle seems like it would encompass diet with how and what you eat has both cultural and regional variations. Are you as confused as I am? Let us proceed.

Today there are hundreds of books dealing with 'diet' promoted as healthy or functional ways to eat that often conflict with a basic dietary lifestyle that an individual or group may traditionally consume. It often is at variance with what is or was regularly consumed (Webster's first definition). In this usage, diet has now been re-defined as eating and consuming food that is NOT in line with what was 'regularly consumed' so it is a behavioral change. Now that impacts our typical way of eating that was defined as lifestyle. Boy, what a mess.

So, are we talking diet or are we talking lifestyle? Wait, if you read a 'diet book' it often refers to a defined period of time to eat in a different manner. Diet now seems to be a temporary way of eating and closer relates to Webster's version three of the definition of 'diet'. In this way then the 'diet' is temporary and not part of the lifestyle of the individual (or group) and not typical as part of the way of life previously experienced. Usually associated with a goal/objective of losing weight or to address a medical condition that may be remediated by this change in diet/lifestyle. So, is diet and lifestyle now the same thing? Only in terms of this temporary span of time it seems.

We now have a temporary eating pattern that impacts both diet and lifestyle so is it still a diet and is it still part of a lifestyle for the individual or group? It seems not to be the case; so, shouldn't we define a different term to refer to this temporary way of obtaining nourishment that is neither part of the person or group's regular eating pattern or consistent with their lifestyle or way of living as culturally defined?

Or, should we coin a term to replace the word diet as it has been so badly compromised that it no longer has any real/true meaning? Has it become so bastardized as to become a useless term? I think so. The word 'diet' has been so misused and abused as to be virtually meaningless. I have a suggestion for a suitable replacement term in the English language, how about Lifestylediet?

A new noun definition that truly defines how a one lives and eats on a regular, long-term basis. It combines two of the existing words into a more meaningful one that better defines the way one obtains nourishment on a regular basis for the rest of their life (or at least until the next major shift in eating pattern).

Lifestylediet is truly all about what you watch, listen to, read and your friends. Be mindful of all the things you put into your body, emotionally, intellectually, spiritually and physically!

Whole Food Plant Based Lifestylediet

Why Plant-Based? Why not? Whole Plant Foods are complete with all their rich natural complement of nutrients, vitamins and minerals. They have not been highly processed nor do they contain synthetic, artificial or irradiated ingredients. They are not genetically modified (non-GMO) to contain pesticide components that have undetermined impacts on the human organism. Whenever possible, *Whole Foods 4 Healthy Living* recommends purchasing "organically grown" foods, since they not only promote your health, but also the health of our planet.

Plant-Based Cuisine encompasses more than just avoiding meat, fish, dairy and eggs. While difficult for many it is pretty darn easy to do these days. There have been many advances in food preparation techniques and new ingredients not available just a few years ago. Now, with new kitchen chemistry and techniques, combined with unique combinations of spices, ingredients and textures you can learn how to prepare almost ALL of those delicious meals you have enjoyed all your life.

Sometimes the most elegant solution is the simplest. Why develop heart disease? Cancer? Diabetes? The epidemic of chronic, degenerative disease that is sweeping the western world can not only be stopped, it can be reversed. The power lies in the hands of the consumer, in the choices we make about what to put on our plates.

Meat and dairy are produced by large corporate food systems that inject the animals with an assortment of drugs, growth hormones, antibiotics and so on. The animals are fed a variety of foodstuffs that are not natural to the animals normal/natural condition. These unnatural foods combined with the drugs and hormones used make meat, fish, dairy and eggs of questionable nutritional value. The massive amounts of antibiotics used in animal farming plus the over-prescribing of antibiotics by 'doctors' has caused the emergence of Superbugs that are resistant to use and pose a significant health risk to humans!

The end result of much of this is that we have a plentiful food supply that may not be all that good for us! Naturally and organically grown whole foods are becoming more plentiful. This is due to the awakening of the American Consumer and the realization that some of our food supply may in fact be harmful.

As with any other dietary change (if this is a major change for you) let us know of any allergies or food sensitivities and/or health conditions you may have. We do not offer nutritional advice or medical counseling but help you migrate/evolve/develop your Plant-Based Lifestyle, by learning how to prepare delicious meals with plant-based whole foods. Please consult your medical professional if this is a dramatic change from your normal lifestyle.

Alternate Diets

I would be remiss if I failed to mention alternate diets and yes, lifestyles. There are many but I will try to adhere to the most popular.

The Art of Healing

Mediterranean Diet - The Mediterranean diet recommends filling your plate with fresh fruits, vegetables, nuts and legumes, with moderate portions of fish and shellfish for protein. Unlike the recommended Whole Food Plant Based Lifestylediet, this diet includes cheeses and other dairy, egg and meat consumption.

Vegetarian Diet – Like the Mediterranean, this diet recommends consuming vegetables, fruits, grains, legumes nuts and seeds. It also includes dairy and egg consumption.

Pescatarian – This diet includes the consumption of fish, dairy and eggs but excludes the consumption of more traditional animal/meat items.

Ketogenic Diet – Is a low carb, high fat diet. The ketogenic diet is based on the principle that by depleting the body of carbohydrates, which are its primary source of energy, you can force the body to burn fat for fuel, thereby maximizing weight loss. This diet we consider very unhealthy as it can promote arterial/heart disease if endured over long periods of time. While it can be very beneficial for select medical conditions it should only be undertaken under medical **supervision.**

There are many more diets out there and many have come/gone over the years/decades. For instance, there was once a popular diet called the Adkins dict, a popular low-carbohydrate eating plan popular in the 70's. This diet limited consumption of fiber-rich food that often led to nutrient imbalance and causing intestinal issues.

People who embark on these 'diet programs' most often view them as a temporary thing that they can lose weight or reverse a metabolic disorder; but seldom as a

The Art of Healing

component of the lifestyle change. This is why most ultimately fail in the long term.

That is one of the reasons we have coined the term Lifestylediet as it better defines a way of living, long term and impacting your current and future wellbeing.

Healing the Entire Human Being

We have covered many modalities and approaches to maintaining and/or restoring the Human Body to a Systems Balance that is called 'Health'. This Gestalt of the Human Being is often referred to as 'being healthy'. This state of have all the body/mind systems in full balance and synchronicity is, for many, a very difficult state to achieve and even more difficult to maintain.

It is often the stated goal of many practitioners to help the patient achieve this goal by means a variety of protocols, treatments and, in many cases, by the application/use of unnatural drugs, surgeries and/or radiation.

The typical refusal to even consider alternative modes of healing or therapies to treat or restore the patient to a state of

The Art of Healing

homeostasis and synchronicity is an abomination that represents the current state of accepted modern medicine.

This is compounded by the fact that most insurance companies will only consider only a few of the alternate therapies, such as acupuncture, for certain conditions/cases.

Not a single insurance carrier/company that we are aware even considers nutrition/diet as a factor in the reimbursable catalogue of treatments. While a few corporations have adopted a more supportive approach to maintaining employee health by sponsoring programs in nutrition, exercise, health fairs and more; they are few and far between.

In the end it always comes down to the words "Physician, heal thyself" from Luke 4:23, as it may bring realization that our own illnesses or troubles can only be dealt with if we, the patient, assume a much more active role in our own health, wellness and

The Art of Healing

longevity. We cannot depend on others, as they have proven over many decades to be incapable of actually doing much for the individual's out of balance systems (both physical and mental).

Taking a more pro-active role in doing research on our or your loved one's condition, seeking alternative modalities of care and support can often prove to be an excellent way to restore the overall balance; the Gestalt we call Health!

This presentation is intended to not be an answer or cure, but an Exposé to make you aware of the many options that are available to treat the source of the symptoms of an unbalanced human body and restore the gestalt of the human being.

****

Thanks, you for your attention. I and Chef Nancy work with people from all over the

The Art of Healing

planet and offer counseling support services. We support ZOOM conferencing as well as have a presence on many social media sites.

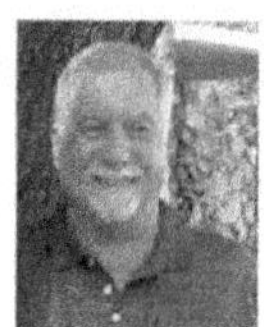
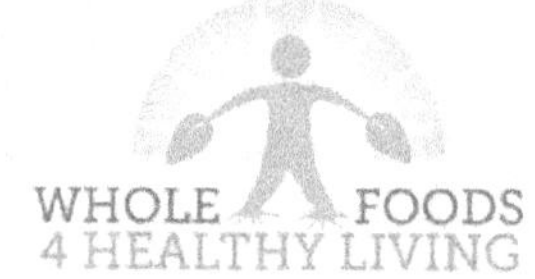

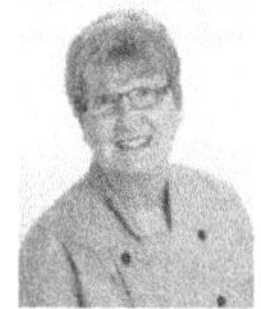

Skip Stein, BS ~ Nancy Stein, PBNC
Lifestyle Counselors, Authors & Speakers
Plant Based Lifestyle Consulting
https://health-healing.wf4hl.com/
Counseling@wfpbls.com Cell:.407.683.6816